Disclaimer:

Always consult with your doctor before starting a new lifestyle change.

Contents

The Steps to Winning

In a journal or on a scratch paper write these steps down. Keep it somewhere you will see it every day.

Steps to winning:

1. What's your reason for making a change in your life?

2. Your personal trigger foods.
    a. We will cover this later in the book.

3. Track it every day what you eat and drink.

4. Share with a friend.

5. What's your attitude today? You don't determine your future, you determine your habits and your habits determine your future.

Acknowledgments

Welcome to my life. I honestly have the best day ever, everyday!

First off, I am so blessed and humbled to be sharing this book with you. I am truly living the life I've dreamed and thought of in my mind. So, first and foremost, *thank you* for reading this book.

How do you say thank you to the people in your life that made you the person whom you've become? For me it would be my wife, my daughter, my mom and dad, my siblings, friends, teachers, coworkers, random people I've met, and spiritual leaders. I could write a whole book on the people I'm thankful for, but let me tell you about the two closest people in my life.

Thank you to my wife. If it wasn't for her, I would have never thought of writing this book. She is the most amazing person on this planet! She is the reason I'm successful in this life. I'm truly blessed to have married her. She was, and still is my dream girl.

Now, here's a little background on my wife Heather. She is such a driven person. When she makes up her mind she is hell bent on getting that project or goal done. She keeps me motivated and I am grateful to have her in my life. I sometimes pinch myself because I cannot believe I'm married to such an amazing person, inside and out. She has always believed in me and trusted my decisions in our life. So, with that support I am here writing *our* first book about not only changing your body, but transforming *you* into the best person you can be!

I also need to thank my daughter for being such a loving and overall good kid. I love you, Boo, for all that you have become, but most of all for just being you! Bryndon, you taught me a very important lesson in life, "If you don't get something your first time around don't quit; *you* must move forward and work harder to get what you want." I'm proud that you made your goal of being a school cheerleader, but more important, that you learned if you don't succeed the first time you must press on. You will go far in life because you have no limits in life. I'm so proud of you! -Love Dad.

The Reason to Move Forward
and
Change Your Life

Please read this chapter closely with your heart and mind. If you do not relate to this chapter or have not gotten to this place in your life then this isn't for you.

I pose some questions for you: Why should I make a change in my life? Why would I make a commitment? Why do I want to lose weight so badly? Is the reason bigger than myself? Well, we are about to answer those questions, but first a quick story about one change I made in my life.

When I was 30 years old I was an outside salesperson working for a large steel distributer. I had a boss that micromanaged me.

One particular day he called me at 7:00 a.m. (I had left that day at 5:00 a.m. to meet a client two hours from my house). He asked "Where are you? I need you to come into the office to go over some inventory issues." I explained I had left early this morning and was nowhere near the office.

This next part is important. He made me feel like crap. I felt like he didn't care about me or the efforts I was making. I was frustrated and felt like he was watching me every second and I hated my job.

I pulled over and started to cry because right there I knew I had to make a change in my life and I hated the position I was in. It was fear that was driving me that day. I knew I couldn't just quit. I had a mortgage, a baby girl and a wife to support. I hit bottom that morning. Bottom, to me, was saying, "Enough is enough!" I had to change my direction in life. I had to find myself again.

Right there off I15 in Payson, Utah I found the answer; it was staring at me right in the face. I needed to pay my house off. I didn't make a lot of money and still owed $170,000 on my mortgage. So, I made a commitment to myself that day by saying every raise I get from this day forward I will use this to pay down the mortgage. Exactly seven years later that became a reality.

"Yahoo, it worked!" I cried again, but not because of stress. Instead, it was because I found a system that worked. I call it "The Reason for the Change."

Some people call it "finding your bottom." Whatever bottom means to you, you need to have a reason. A person's deep-down reason to make a change. Without this reason you will not be committed to make that change in your life.

***

Later in my life, right before I turned 40, I was on a cruise with some customers. My wife and I were lying out on the top deck of this Carnival cruise ship enjoying the sunshine, when a friend and customer came up to me and said, "Wow JJ (my nickname), I've never seen you with a gut before." It was embarrassing. That comment hit me hard.

Let me clarify something about this friend, he is a great person with a heart of gold and says things the way they need to be said. Direct, to the point, and no B.S. Those are the kind of friends I love to have in my life.

When we got home from our cruise I was in our kitchen and happened to have my shirt off that day. My 10-year-old daughter, Bryndon, came up to me and said, "Dad you have 'man boobs.'" This was another significant chapter in my life.

After that, time stopped and I knew I needed to make a change. I needed to shift directions because after those two comments I knew I wanted to be better. I hit another bottom in my life. I didn't like the way I looked or the lack of confidence I had so I needed to make a change.

***

I was watching a P90X® commercial on TV and knew that was what I needed. First of all, I needed structure, a plan. I knew my will power was up for the challenge. Well, within 90 days I lost 30 pounds and had gotten into great shape. I continued this path for two years, repeated the program and achieved extreme results.

But I kept falling backwards with my weight loss because I overate. I know now that my Trigger Foods, what I like to call "forbidden fruit," were making me fail.

What is a Trigger Food?

Here's where the work comes in. I need you to get a clean piece of paper and start thinking about your trigger foods; write them down. Memorize this this list because you will need it later.

What is a trigger food? Well, it's any food that makes you want to continue to eat and not stop. So, for example, trigger foods for me include pizza, salted nuts, Oreo's, cake, brownies, sweets, candy bars, and chips and salsa. I can't just have one.

I need you, over the next five days, to think about your trigger foods and write them down on a piece of paper. This task is important, it will lay out the road map for your future to help you understand what to watch and stay away from. Am I saying that these types of foods to you and me are like an alcoholic drink to an alcoholic? Yes, yes I am. This list you are about to write are your "forbidden fruits."

Now don't say to yourself, "Man this guy is nuts. I'm not cutting out cake on my daughter's birthday or on my birthday! He's crazy!" That is not what I am saying. You need to be aware of what makes you over eat and makes you gain weight; that's what I'm saying. So, let's continue with this list.

These are my personal trigger foods:

- Pizza
- Nuts
- Cookies
- Bread
- Oreo's
- Cake
- Brownies
- Sweets
- Candy Bars
- Chips and Salsa
- Deep fried *anything*
- Chicken fried rice
- Buffalo wings

Big bags of any of these foods in my house or car will cause me to overeat. When I am able to stay away from these foods my odds of achieving my goal increase dramatically.

***

Now let's discuss beverages.
I suggest you remove the listed beverages from your diet to help you achieve your goal.

Alcohol:
When you drink any alcohol, it drives your senses, or as I call them "uncontrollable urges to eat crap."

Carbonation:
Carbonation causes bloating. While trying to lose weight and change your lifestyle consuming carbonated beverages can make it more difficult to get to your goal weight.

Caffeine:
Limit the intake of caffeine. Your adrenal glands will thank you. Caffeine can also result in low energy levels, headaches, and other health issues.

Bad foods (or drinks) are typically trigger foods that cause you to start going down the wrong road. So, my advice is to not drink at all through my program, not even a cheat day. You will see life and other people in a different light, I can promise you that.

Going back to your list, for five days you must have this list by your side. Keep it by your bed at night and at your desk at work. I want you to continue to think about your trigger foods. *What are they? Why do I eat them? Where do I buy them? Who buys them for me?*

What are your trigger foods?

1.

2.

3.

4.

5.

Once you have written down your trigger foods I need you to share this list with your family, friends, co-workers or whomever. They need to understand that you are no longer going to keep these foods in your home.

What are bad foods?

"In my personal opinion, bad foods are anything that is processed at a plant or has an expiration date on the label. It was once said, 'if it doesn't come from the ground or doesn't have mother don't eat it.'" –Jillian Michaels

I fully agree with this statement.[1]

What does it mean to eat clean?

If you read the above statement you will see clean eating means eating any food that has not been processed at a plant. Adding chemicals to your food is never good for your body.

Ways to eat clean

Protein:

Protein is an essential part of every diet. Your body needs protein to stay strong and healthy.

---

[1] Note: All bread is processed and this is not allowed while you are following the T rigger Foods plan.

It also aids in building muscle, maintaining a healthy weight, and keeping you full by increasing metabolism. There many different sources of protein, including seafood, lean meat, poultry, beans, and nuts.

It is recommended that you eat one gram of protein per pound of body weight if you are trying to build lean muscle. Consuming protein suppresses those carb trigger food impulses. Below I have listed some suggested sources of protein.

SEAFOOD

Seafood is a great protein because it is low in fat but high in necessary nutrients, including omega-3, magnesium, and vitamins A and D. Some suggested seafood includes:

- Catfish
- Clams
- Cod
- Crab
- Crayfish
- Flounder
- Halibut
- Herring
- Lobster
- Mussels
- Octopus
- Oysters
- Pollock
- Salmon
- Scallops
- Sea bass
- Shrimp
- Snapper
- Squid
- Swordfish
- Trout
- Tuna

Lean Meats

Lean meats contain less fat and lower amounts of saturated fats. You can identify lean cuts by the label. Look for cuts labeled "loin" or "round." Lean meats include (organic and grass fed):

- Beef
- Bison
- Ham
- Lamb
- Pork
- Veal
- Venison

Poultry

Poultry contains essential amino acids and a low amount of fat. It is an ideal substitute for fatty meats and doesn't break the bank. Poultry (organic is ideal) includes:

- Chicken
- Duck
- Free range eggs
- Goose
- Ground chicken and turkey
- Turkey

BEANS AND LENTILS

Beans and lentils are a great protein substitute and are high in fiber, which meats are not. Beans and lentils include:

- Bean burgers
- Black beans
- Black eyed peas
- Chickpeas
- Kidney beans
- Lentils
- Lima beans
- Navy beans
- Pinto beans
- Soy beans
- Split peas
- White beans

NUTS AND SEEDS

Nuts and seeds are loaded with nutrients and can be a great snack to keep on hand.

- Almonds
- Cashews
- Hazelnuts
- Mixed nuts
- Peanuts
- Peanut butter
- Pecans
- Pistachios
- Pumpkin seeds
- Sesame seeds
- Sunflower seeds
- Walnuts

SUPPLEMENTS

When consuming a protein drink I recommend brands that are high in casein and low in sugar and carbs.

Carbs:

Carbohydrates provide your body with energy. However, there are good carbs and bad carbs. Like discussed earlier in Jillian Michael's quote, it needs to come from the ground and not be processed.

For this plan to work, you will need to cut out carbs like bread and pasta and stick with natural carbs. Below is a list of suggested natural carbs that will help you lose weight and feel great.

- Asparagus
- Beans
- Broccoli
- Brown rice
- Carrots
- Green
- Kale
- Lentils
- Mushrooms
- Nuts
- Oats and oatmeal
- Potatoes
- Pumpkin
- Quinoa
- Seaweed
- Seeds
- Snow peas
- Spinach
- Sweet potato
- Tomatoes
- Yams
- Zucchini

Fruits:

Fruits are an important part of a well-balanced diet. They are naturally low in sodium and fat and provide many essential nutrients including fiber, vitamin C, and potassium.

- Apples
- Bananas
- Berries
- Lemons
- Limes
- Mango

- Oranges
- Peaches
- Pineapple
- Plums
- Watermelon

Good fats:

There is a difference between good fats and bad fats. Good fats are an important part of your diet. They provide essential fatty acids and vitamins to keep our bodies fueled. Below are two different types of good fats, monounsaturated and polyunsaturated.

Monounsaturated fats

In chemistry, "mono" means one. So, a monounsaturated fat has one unsaturated chemical bond. This type of fat is typically found in oils and foods such as canola oil, olive oil, and avocados and will start to solidify if refrigerated.

- Avocados
- Canola oil
- Nuts
- Olive oil
- Olives

- Peanut butter
- Peanut oil
- Sesame oil
- Sunflower oil

Polyunsaturated fats

Back to chemistry, "poly" means more than one. So, a polyunsaturated fat has many unsaturated chemical bonds. This can typically be found in sesame oil, sunflower seeds, and fatty fish.

- Corn oil
- Fatty fish
- Flaxseed
- Pumpkin seeds
- Safflower oil
- Sesame

- Soybean oil
- Sunflower oil
- Walnuts
- Soymilk
- Tofu

Condiments, herbs and spices:

Condiments, herbs and spices add flavor to a meal. However, many may include unnecessary added fats, sugars, sodium, etc. Below are a few recommended condiments, herbs and spices for this program.

- Apple cider vinegar
- Balsamic vinegar
- Black pepper
- Cayenne pepper
- Dijon mustard
- Fresh garlic
- Fresh ginger
- Fresh herbs
- Mrs. Dash seasonings
- Sea salt
- Seeded mustard
- White wine vinegar

Eating Schedule

How many times a day should you eat? It is best to eat at least 4-6 times a day to keep you from becoming hungry and turning to your trigger foods.

My ideal eating times include:

1. Within one hour of waking up
2. After working out
3. Snack
4. Lunch
5. Snack
6. Dinner

Attitude Adjustment

OK, take another pause and ask yourself a few simple questions.

If I wanted to be rich who would I talk to? Someone living on the streets or Bill Gates? The obvious choice would be Bill Gates.

If I wanted to be happy who would I talk to? A negative person or positive person?

If I wanted to be healthy and fit who would I talk to? Obviously someone who is in great shape.

They have the skills, discipline and knowledge to get you from point A to point B. You are a product of your surroundings. I'm helping you keep these trigger foods out of your reach, for now, and after 90 days it will become a habit.

Who are your friends?

This is pretty simple. Write down your five closest friends. Who are they and are they taking the same path you want to take?

I truly believe that you need to be very careful who your favorite five people are in your life (excluding family). These friends are either going to lift you up or bring you down. Rid yourself of the friends in your life that are not going to support you in your goals. If you surround yourself with positive and successful people, you can be positive and successful too.

The Attitude Adjustment

A positive attitude is the most important step in this whole process. Without it your chances of reaching your goals diminish.

Now, I want you to think about what makes you happy. Is it your friends? Well, you need to have more friends like this in your life. Surround yourself with successful people. This doesn't mean people with money. Money doesn't make you successful. It's a person's character, word, and actions towards others. I want this for you.

So, what type of attitude do the people you hang out have?

The Circle of Life

As you may have already figured out, this is not just about you having a great body, which you will receive if you follow my plan, but about your circle of life.

Image that you have six circles around your body. One circle is your health and fitness, one is finances, one is spiritual, one is family, one is giving oneself to others, and one is your piece of mind. When anyone of these circles is in disarray they tend to screw up your "circle of life."

So, we need to continue to work on all these circles in our lives. When you get your health in check, I will challenge you to continue to learn and read. Keep improving as you grow in this program.

***

To be successful at a lifestyle change you need to have a good reason to change, a true deep down drive to keep you going every day. Your thoughts, if pushed in the right direction, will help you accomplish anything you want in life.

My wife and I talk constantly about the positive things that are going on in our life. How blessed we are, the direction we are heading, the wonderful friends we have in our lives. It's amazing to see how great our life has become and it truly keeps getting better. I always tell my wife "the best is yet to come" and it's true our life does get better by the day, month and year.

Are you going to have negative thoughts once in a while? Of course, but you can learn how to get rid of them. If you can control it, then fix it. If you can't you must let it go. It's that simple.

The 21-Days to a Lifestyle Change

This is a lifestyle change, not a diet. It takes 21 days to make something a habit. Trigger Foods wants to help you with those first 21 days and we hope you find the strength to continue on with your lifestyle change.

Today is your day, cease it and let's get started.

***

A few things to consider before we begin:

1. I want you to take two pictures of yourself-a front view and a side view. Then after the 90 days I want you take the same pictures. I will then ask you to please submit your results so others can see your accomplishments.

    Submit photos to marketing@yourtf.com.

2. Let's calculate how many calories you need to maintain your current weight, and then adjust. I suggest searching for a calorie counter online. Many of these tools will have your goal weight.

I recommend you have this when tracking your food daily so you know if you are winning or losing.

3. Review the section on eating clean.

    Refer to the quote by Jillian Michael's at the beginning of this
    book.

4. Track your daily food intake.

    It is important that you track everything you eat throughout
    your 90 day plan. This will allow you to see where you are going and identify what you can improve on. It takes discipline, but the results will make it worthwhile.[2]

5. What will change with your body?

    As you change what you eat your body will reward you. You will begin to see results within the first week of clean eating and exercising. You will notice a change in your mind as well as your body. You can do this.

6. What is a cheat meal?

---

[2] There are plenty of apps and websites out there that will track and record your calories for you.

A cheat meal will replenish the glycogen storage back into the muscle and in return help with energy and blood sugar balance. The extra calories from a cheat meal will speed up your metabolism as much as 9%.

The Plan

The Trigger Foods plan allows you one cheat meal a week. This can be anytime during the week, but may not exceed one meal. We suggest you completely removed your trigger foods from your diet for these 21 days. It will get easier and you will eventually stop craving them. You will learn how to eat them in moderation.

While on this plan make sure you eat every couple hours. If you are hungry, do not starve yourself. Pick up a vegetable, fruit or protein and stay away from those trigger foods.

***

Based on your weight and your goals, here is a typical 21-day eating plan for the beginner.

Tip: Plan your meals every day. This will help you stick to the plan. A great way to do this is to cook all your meals for the week on Sunday. Figure out what you are eating every meal of the week. Put your snacks (veggies, fruit, nuts, etc.) in snack size storage bags so they are already prepared for you. This will ensure fast food and convenient stores don't plan your food intake.

Make sure you stop eating an hour and a half before bed so your body has time to digest your food intake.

These are just suggestions. If you need to add more to your portion, add more. Just don't overeat. Listen to your body. Once you incorporate clean eating your body will crave this new way of fueling it.

Sample recipes in the index.

Example #1-One Week Sample Meal Plan
Carb Cycling Meal Plan
Based on a Monday-Sunday week.

Tip: Eat every couple hours to keep your metabolism going. Drink plenty of water while doing this plan. Eight cups of water is recommended, but you may need more depending on your day.

MONDAY: HIGH CARB DAY

Breakfast:

- ¾ cup oatmeal (measured dry)
- ½ cup mixed berries (can be frozen but not sweetened)
- 1 tsp. of Truvia or agave (if needed)

Snack:

- orange

Lunch:

- ¾ cup brown rice
- ½ a mango, sliced
- 6 oz. grilled chicken
- 1 cup green beans

Snack:

- apple

Dinner:

- ¾ cup quinoa
- 6 oz. white fish
- 1 cup steamed broccoli

TUESDAY: HIGH CARB DAY

Breakfast:

- spelt bread & egg white French toast
- fresh strawberries or
- 1/8 cup sugar free maple syrup

Snack:

- 1 fresh pear

Lunch:

- turkey wrap with lettuce (no tortilla or br ead)
    - 6 oz. turkey
    - Romaine lettuce leaves
- mustard and plain yogurt for condiments

Snack:

- a protein bar (I like Quest bars-beware of sugar and carb content)

Dinner:

- ¾ cup brown rice
- 6 oz. ground turkey
- ½ diced green pepper
- 1 cup of mushrooms
- 1 cup green beans

WEDNESDAY: HIGH PROTEIN DAY

Breakfast:

- 5-egg white scramble with onions and gre en peppers
- 2 tsp. low sodium salsa

Snack:

- can of tuna in water
- diced pickles and onion
- 3 Tbsp. 0% Greek yogurt

Lunch:

- Heather's Tuna Salad (recipe in index)

Snack:

- 4 hardboiled egg whites

Dinner:

- 6 oz. grilled chicken
- 1 cup steamed broccoli and cauliflower

THURSDAY: HIGH PROTEIN DAY

Breakfast:

- 5 scrambled egg whites with spinach
- 6 oz. 0% Greek yogurt

Snack:

- Protein bar

Lunch:

- 6 oz. chicken
- 3 cups of mixed greens
- Red wine vinegar for dressing

Snack:

- 1 can of chicken breast w/diced onion an d pickle
- 6 oz. 0% Greek yogurt

Dinner:

- 6 oz. lean steak
- 1 cup asparagus

FRIDAY: MIX OF CARBS, PROTEIN AND FAT

Breakfast:

- ½ cup oatmeal (measured dry)
- 1 cup mixed berries
- 2 scrambled eggs (with yolk) with mushrooms, tomatoes and spinach

Snack:

- 12 bite-size carrots
- 2 Tbsp. hummus

Lunch:

- 6 oz. chicken
- 3 cups mixed greens
- ½ lemon squeezed over for dressing

Snack:

- 2 6-in celery
- 2 Tbsp. almond butter

Dinner:

- 6 oz. chicken breast
- jicama slices
- 4 oz. sweet potato

SATURDAY: MIX OF CARBS, PROTEIN AND FAT

Breakfast:

- ½ cup steel cut oats
- ½ cup raspberries
- 2 hardboiled eggs

Snack:

- 12 almonds

Lunch:

- open faced turkey sandwich on spelt brea d
  - 6 oz. turkey
- hummus spread

Snack:

- protein bar

Dinner:

- 6 oz. salmon
- 2 cups asparagus

SUNDAY: MIX OF CARBS, PROTEIN AND FAT

Breakfast:

- 3 egg omelet (with yolk) w/avocado
- 2 tsp. low sodium salsa
- 1 slice of toasted spelt bread

Snack:

- 2 Tbsp. almond butter

Lunch:

- 4 oz. ground lean hamburger in romaine l ettuce leaves w/ tomatoes

Snack:

- 12 baby carrots
- 2 Tbsp. hummus

Dinner:

- Broiled White Fish (recipe in index)
- 2 cups green beans

Example #2-One Week Sample Meal Plan[3]
Protein Kick Start Meal Plan

<u>MONDAY</u>

Breakfast:

- 5 egg white omelet w/mushrooms, peppers and onions
- 1 banana

Snack:

- *See 100 calorie snack list in index*

Lunch:

- chicken salad w/peppers, mushrooms, and onions (no cheese)
  - 6 oz. chicken
- oil and vinegar as dressing

Snack:

- *See 100 calorie snack list in index*

Dinner:

- 6 oz. fresh fish
- 1 cup any veggie

Late night snack:

---

[3] You can eat 5-6 times a day, depending on your goal and caloric intake.

- ½ cup 2% low-fat cottage cheese

TUESDAY

Breakfast:

- 5 egg whites w/spinach
- 1 cup berries

Snack:

- *See 100 calorie snack list in index*

Lunch:

- chicken lettuce sandwich w/ tomatoes and onions
- Use mustard as your condiment

Snack:

- *See 100 calorie snack list in index*

Dinner:

- veggie stir fry w/mushrooms, peppers, onions, tomatoes, and spinach
- olive oil to cook

Late night snack:

- ½ cup 2% low-fat cottage cheese

WEDNESDAY

Breakfast:

- Spinach Onion Super Scramble (recipe in index)

- 1 banana

Snack:

- *See 100 calorie snack list in index*

Lunch:

- chicken, walnut and veggie salad
    - 6 oz. grilled chicken
- 2 Tbsp. raspberry vinaigrette

Snack:

- *See 100 calorie snack list in index*

Dinner:

- 6 oz. chicken
- ½ cup brown rice
- 1 cup veggies

Late Night snack:

- ½ cup 2% low-fat cottage cheese

THURSDAY

Breakfast:

- ½ cup oatmeal (measured dry)
- 12 almonds

Snack:

- *See 100 calorie snack list in index*

Lunch:

- 6 oz. fresh salmon
- 1 cup veggies

Snack:

- *See 100 calorie snack list in index*

Dinner:

- 6 oz. chicken breast
- 1 cup veggies

Late Night Snack:

- ½ cup 2% low-fat cottage cheese

FRIDAY

Breakfast:

- 5 egg white omelet w/mushrooms, peppers, and onions[4]
- 1 banana

Snack:

- *See 100 calorie snack list in index*

Lunch:

- chicken, walnut and veggie salad
    - 6 oz. grilled chicken
- 2 Tbsp. raspberry vinaigrette

Snack:

- *See 100 calorie snack list in index*

Dinner:

- 6 oz. lean steak
- ½ cup brown rice
- 1 cup veggies

---

[4] Try mixing it up with other veggies. Tomatoes, asparagus, and spinach are also great choices to add to your morning omelet.

Late Night snack:

- ½ cup 2% low-fat cottage cheese

SATURDAY

Breakfast:

- 5 egg white omelet w/mixed veggies
- 1 banana

Snack:

- *See 100 calorie snack list in index*

Lunch:

- chicken lettuce wrap w/tomatoes and onions
- mustard

Snack:

- *See 100 calorie snack list in index*

Dinner:

- 6 oz. fresh tilapia
- 1 cup veggies
- 4 oz. sweet potato

Late Night snack:

- ½ cup 2% low-fat cottage cheese

SUNDAY

Breakfast:

- Spinach Onion Super Scramble (recipe in index)
- 1 of banana

Snack:

- See 100 calorie snack list

Lunch:

- chicken salad w/peppers, mushrooms, and onions (no cheese)
  - 6 oz. chicken
- oil and vinegar as dressing

Snack:

- See 100 calorie snack list

Dinner:

- 6 oz. fresh fish
- 1 cup any veggie

Late night snack:

- ½ cup 2% low-fat cottage cheese

***

JJ's special note: *Seven steps to a new you*

1. Reason it. Have a true reason for changing yourself.

   I want you to post it were you will be able to see it at any time during the day.

Also post a picture of what that change looks like to you.

2. Plan it. Prepare your food list first thing when you wake up or the night before. Planning ahead will ensure you win today. Don't worry about the past or the future today is the only day that matters.

3. Journal it. At the end of each day write down everything you ate. Then every Sunday I want you to share this list with someone. This will keep you accountable for your actions.

4. Think it. As Aristotle states, "We are what we repeatedly do. Excellence, then, is not an act, but a habit."

5. Live it. Keep focused on your goals.

6. Share it. Share your success with friends.

Exercise

Exercise three to five times a week for a minimum of 30 minutes each workout. Add weight training or Pilates two to three days a week for 30 minutes. Abdominal focused exercises one day a week for 10 minutes is also recommended.

Make sure to add cardio to your workouts if you are trying to lose weight. Cardio keeps your heart rate up and helps burn fat.

For workout ideas visit www.yourtf.com for how to's and tips.

Track It

Tracking what you eat will keep you accountable to meet your fitness and attitude goals. It is imperative that you either write down in a journal or use a fitness and nutrition tracker app[5] to keep track of every meal and work out.

I also would like you to make a note every day in your journal (or app) on how you feel that day. Good or bad.

Share your stories with us. Follow us on social media to see other success stories and to let your story be heard.

---

[5] I personally use MyFitnessPal. It allows you to invite friends to it and keeps you accountable not only to yourself but to your accountability partners.

What's Next?

You now have the knowledge, plan, and road map to get you where you need to go. Only you can make the difference. So, take action right now and change your life!

Let's recap the highlights.

1. Have a strong reason to make a change.
2. Track your trigger foods for five days, write them down and memorize them.
3. Attitude: what are you thinking? Do you have forward positive thinking?
4. Whom are you hanging out with? Are they taking you up or down?
5. Plan your eating week to win.
6. Plan your exercise for the week stick to it.
7. Track your progress. Any app on your smart phone that tracks food is great, but simply keeping a journal will also hold you accountable.
8. Cardio/weight lifting. Three days a week and 30 minutes per day of cardio/weight lifting to get the best results.

Congratulations on finishing this plan! Trigger Foods is all about lifestyle choices. Now that you have reached your goal, keep it up!

Please make sure to submit your before and after pictures to marketing@yourtf.com.

Index

Recipes

Spinach Onion Super Scramble

<u>INGREDIENTS</u>

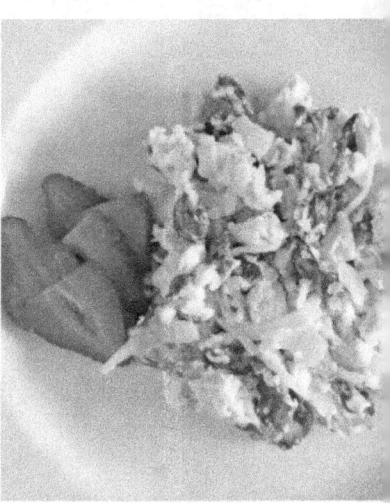

1 large egg

4 large egg whites

1 pinch sea salt

1 pinch ground black pepper

1 tsp. Olive oil

½ cup fresh baby spinach

½ cup chopped white onions

<u>DIRECTIONS</u>

- Combine egg, egg whites, salt and pepper in medium bowl; whisk to blend. Set aside.
- Heat oil in medium nonstick skillet over medium-low heat.
- Add spinach and onion; cook, stirring frequently, for 2 to 3 minutes.

- Add egg mixture, cook, stirring frequently, for 2 to 3 minutes, or until eggs are cooked through.

Heather's Tuna Salad

INGREDIENTS

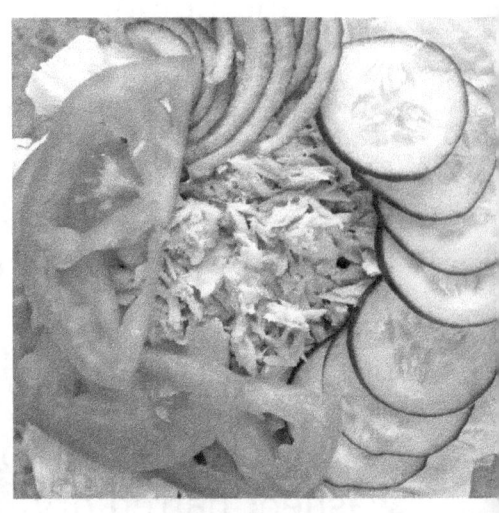

¾ cup canned light tuna in water, drained (approximately 4.5 oz.)

1 tsp. extra-virgin olive oil

1 Tbsp. fresh lemon juice

1 cup romaine lettuce

¼ cup sliced cucumber

¼ cup sliced red radishes

¼ cup cherry tomatoes, cut in half

¼ cup thinly sliced red onion

Red wine vinegar

DIRECTIONS

- Combine tuna, oil, and lemon juice, mix well.
- Place lettuce on a large serving plate.
- Top with cucumber, radishes, tomatoes, and onion.
- Top with tuna, drizzle with vinegar.

Roasted Cauliflower Bowl

INGREDIENTS

4 cups cauliflower florets, washed, patted dry

4 tsp. olive oil

1 tsp sea salt

¼ tsp granulated garlic (Optional)

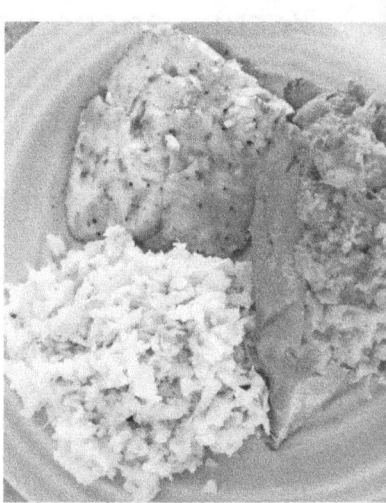

2 Tbsp. low-sodium organic veggie broth

DIRECTIONS

- Preheat oven to 400 degree F.
- Place cauliflower on large baking pan.
- Drizzle with oil; toss gently to coat. Season with salt and garlic (optional).

- Bake, stirring halfway through; for 40 to 45 minutes or until tender.
- Place in food processor; add veggie broth. Pulse until smooth.

Broiled White Fish

INGREDIENTS

4 oz. raw white fish fillets (cod, tilapia, sole, etc.)

4 tsp. olive oil

Chopped fresh oregano

Fresh lemon to taste; optional

DIRECTIONS

- Preheat broiler to high.
- Drizzle with oil. Season with fresh chopped oregano.
- Broil fish for about 3 to 5 minutes until fish is opaque and flakes easily when tested with a fork. Squeeze fresh lemon before serving.

Cinnamon Sweet Potato

INGREDIENTS

9 oz. raw sweet potatoes

Ground cinnamon

Ground black pepper

DIRECTIONS

- Preheat oven to 400 degree F.
- Cover a baking pan with aluminum foil. Set aside.
- Scrub sweet potatoes and pierce several times with fork. Bake for 35 to 45 minutes, or until tender.
- Remove sweet potatoes from oven; cool for 15 minutes.
- Place sweet potato flesh in a medium bowl. Sprinkle with cinnamon and pepper, mash until well mixed.

100 Calorie Snack List

2 med kiwi fruits

10 baby carrots and 2 Tbsp. hummus

½ cup 2% cottage cheese

¾ cup Fage' 0% Greek yogurt

1 slice spelt bread

2 stalks celery

1 large hardboiled egg

½ cup raisin bran

1 brown rice cake w/1/2 Tbsp. natural peanut butter

1 medium cucumber

1 string cheese w/½ small apple

2 cups watermelon balls

4 slices turkey rolled up and dipped in 2 tsp. honey mustard

1 small apple sliced and sprinkled w/cinnamon

1 cup red raspberries w/2 Tbsp. plain Fage' 0% Greek yogurt

2 graham cracker squares w/1 tsp. natural peanut butter

15 mini pretzel sticks w/2 Tbsp. fat-free cream cheese

1/3 cup cooked quinoa

3 Tbsp. all-natural granola

9-10 black olives

7 saltine crackers

2 cups air-popped popcorn w/1 tsp. butter

25 peanuts

2 Tbsp. flaxseeds

3 oz. tuna, canned in water

½ cup cantaloupe topped w/½ cup low-fat cottage cheese

1 nectarine

1 fresh pomegranate

7 plain animal crackers

40 Pepperidge Farm gold fish

1 med tomato w/pinch of salt

2 small peaches

1 cup strawberries

30 grapes

1 cup oat cereal (cheerios)

17 pecans

1 can V8

Med grapefruit sprinkled with salt

8 small shrimp w/3 Tbsp. cocktail sauce

1 cup slice zucchini, seasoned to taste

10 cashews

2 Tbsp. sunflower seeds

For more information about Trigger Foods, LLC or the author visit www.yourtf.com or follow us on social media.